Published and distributed by Joseph Bently Black Diamond, AB. T0L 0H0
First Edition

Library and Archives Canada Cataloguing in Publication

Bentley, Joseph, 1983-, author
    The five divisions of stress recovery / by Joseph Bentley.

ISBN 978-0-9951663-0-1 (paperback)

            1. Stress management. 2. Stress (Physiology). 3. Stress
            (Psychology). I. Title.

RA785.B46 2016   155.9'042   C2016-902727-9

Headshot by back cover Erin Wallace Photography
To order books: joseph@josephbentley.info
visit www. www.josephbentley.info
email: joseph@josephbentley.info

The 5 Divisions
of Stress Recovery

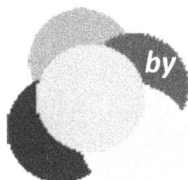

by Joseph Bentley

This book is dedicated to my friends and family; without your support this never would have been possible.

Table of Contents

INTRODUCTION

As far back as I can remember, I have been involved with competitive sports. I swam competitively from the ages of five to twelve, and started to wrestle in grade seven. For the next ten years I competed nationally and internationally as a freestyle wrestler, and finished my career just as I completed my undergraduate degree at the University of Calgary.

By then, my body and my life were both in chaos; I drank heavily (or what college students would call "socially"), slept poorly, my mood would change at the drop of a dime, and chronic injuries left me unable to practice consistently. At the same time, I was experiencing an extremely difficult breakup with my girlfriend, who was also a wrestler. There was no relief from the drama of our split; we shared the same group of friends and were forced to see each other every day at practice.

The stressors in my life had piled up and I was unable to address them. My physical body

had come apart from years as a
wrestler. My mental body was
on empty from the completion of
my undergraduate degree. My
emotional body was completely
shot from the breakup. The
breakup had also shattered me
spiritually, and left me unsure
whom I could trust in my
community. My internal systems
were devastated from alcohol.
My eating habits swung between
restricting food intake to lose
weight for a competition and
eating the way most university
students do—as cheaply and
quickly as possible.

By the end of the fall semester
of school, I felt like my whole life
had fallen apart. The wrestling
room had been my sanctuary,
and a place where I could go to
release excess energy. Now it was
a prison, where my body refused to
move the way I needed it to, and
where I relived the heartache of
my failed relationship.

Graduation from University had
also added the question of what I
would do next in my life. Thinking
of a career path both exhilarated
and terrified me. I would lie awake

*"Get off the
Medical System
and onto the Self
Care System"*
— *Nina Leavins*

at night and question if I was actually passionate enough about Disability Studies to make a career out of it, and why I had gone to university at all.

While all these events unfolded, my family caught only glimpses of my struggles. They might see that I was emotionally upset one day, or walked around the house with a limp the next, but nobody was aware that my life was in chaos.

When I look back, it's easy to see many ways I went wrong, but I was a naive twenty-two-year-old, trying to do my best and failing miserably. I didn't value my health, and because it wasn't a priority, it had fallen by the wayside. I was an athlete, so I assumed I was healthy. But now I slept on a yoga mat—I had allowed my back to become so injured that I couldn't sleep comfortably on a bed.

But there was a lesson that came from this time in my life. When I started to reflect on the breakup, the injuries and the graduation, I asked myself, "Why was that time in my life stressful enough to break me down so much?" I'd had similar life crises before university and they hadn't hit me as hard. I'd had breakups before that didn't hurt as much. And I'd trained just as hard (if not harder) for years without injuries. So what was different about 2006?

I remembered that when I had first started to wrestle, my body had been much more resilient. I would get sore after practice, or tired by the end of the week, but my body would bounce back. Every week I could push it to the limit, and by the end of the weekend I was just as ready to wrestle as I had been the previous Monday—but stronger, faster and more technical. In my early years, I would finish a practice and then do extra workouts. I would push my body to the limit day in and day out. But by the end of my career, I was just happy if I could make it through practice without a new injury. Where had that resiliency gone?

The answer was obvious. Those three events in a short time created an increased load in stress levels that I couldn't handle. The combination of graduation, the

"The time to relax is when you don't have time for it."
– Sydney J. Harris

breakup and my injuries, created the perfect storm of factors that completely wiped me out. But I felt there had to be more–some other part of the puzzle that I couldn't see. It wasn't until years later that I began to realize that stress never leaves; you either recover from it or you don't.

This book evolved from that revelation. If stress is unavoidable, then the effects of how we address and recover from it will impact our health and wellness. This approach to recovery takes some time and effort to implement, but the rewards are profound. In this book, I will help you identify which recovery tools will work for you in your personal and professional life. I found five distinct divisions of stress and recovery that we can use to manage stress more efficiently. I'd like to share this discovery with everyone who feels as though they have too much stress in their lives, and wants to find a way to recover from it more efficiently.

WHAT IS A RECOVERY TOOL?

A recovery tool is anything that you use to help you recover from stress. Just like a regular toolbox you want to make sure you have the right tool for the job. A hammer is a great tool; providing you're hammering in nails. The same can be said of recovery tools; it's important to use the right tool for each of the different divisions of stress and recovery (more on this to come). If you take the time to build your recovery toolbox with a variety of different recovery tools, then you will have an appropriate recovery option for any given situation.

A QUICK LOOK AT STRESS

Stress is an unavoidable reality of life. With our jobs, relationships, commutes and professional schedules, we constantly battle the exhaustive effects of stress on the body.

With friends and family, we talk about how we need to get rid of stress in our lives, to find a better balance between our energy input and output. Sometimes our body feels like a car with an empty gas tank, with no gas station in sight and a distant memory of how nice it used to feel to be fully vibrant and healthy. Our stressors pile up, and with no tools in our toolkit to respond, we start to ask, "When did life get so stressful?"

It's hard to deny that stress can negatively impact your health and wellness. Unfortunately, this only paints the bleak picture that if you have a job, a family, and haven't won the lottery, then you're doomed to a life of low back pain, heart attacks and strokes. But that's not the entire story. There are differences between positive and negative stressors, and our mindset towards them dictates in part how they affect us. If you know that you have the tools and strategies to recover from a stressor, your relationship to it changes. You become more confident that you can use small breaks to your advantage when it comes to stress management; because in reality, not all stress is bad.

The dirty little secret about stress is that it can also propel us to greatness. Stress can cause a mother to lift a car, a community to join closer together, or an athlete to rise to the challenge of competition. Certain types of stress have brought out the best in people, provided they have the resources and proper mindset to handle that stressor appropriately, and the time to recover afterwards.

With that in mind, is stress removal really the answer? How realistic is it to think that we can ever fully remove stress from our lives? After all, there are stressors in our life that provide great rewards. To raise a child may be one of the most stressful decisions a person can make. Yet most parents would never trade

"We can easily manage if we will only take, each day, the burden appointed to it. But the load will be too heavy for us if we carry yesterday's burden over again today, and then add the burden of the morrow before we are required to bear it."
– John Newton

that experience for the world. A job places stressful demands on you, even if it's your dream job. In fact, we usually look for a job that provides some form of challenge, and with challenge comes growth, accompanied by stress. Commuting to and from work can cause massive amounts of stress; this might be the price we pay to live in our desired community, or to work at the job we want.

Then there are the stressors that we simply can't escape. A death in the family, an unexpected expense or a major natural disaster are situations beyond our control. But they are stresses that we may be forced to deal with in our life. And while it would be nice to tell the bank that your account balance is a source of stress, I doubt they would throw a million dollars into your bank account in the name of stress reduction.

There are times in our lives when we need to identify what factors are creating excess stress for us and to take action if possible. There may be work environments, relationships with friends or coworkers, and lifestyle choices where we can make changes. It's incredibly important to be able to identify toxic relationships or environments and move away from them. But in those areas of your life where you can't remove the stress, wouldn't it be nice to feel like you had some control over it's effects on you?

Reframe your thoughts from "How can I have less stress in my life?" to "How can I better recover from the stress in my life?" The tools you will acquire by the end of this book will help you focus on what you can do each day to recover more quickly and completely from stress.

When you have the tools to recover properly from stressors, you have the ability to restructure your relationship to them. Events and situations that once terrified you become less of an issue, because you know you will be able to recover from them afterwards. This is a shift in focus from the common notion that you must avoid as much stress as possible— as we've established, some stressors simply can't be avoided.

Imagine that you have an

"Take rest; a field that has rested gives a bountiful crop."
– Ovid

appointment at the bank to discuss your finances. If you're like me, this evokes a great deal of mental and emotional stress. You may feel judged by the financial advisor about your account balances, or frustrated at your lack of financial savvy. If you decide to cut out all stress, you simply don't go the bank, but you'll also miss out on some potentially valuable advice that could save you a great deal of stress in the long run.

Instead, if you know that the trip to the bank will cause you stress, you can set up recovery opportunities before and after the visit that will minimize the negative impact. Identify your personal recovery tools from mental and emotional stresses, and either incorporate them into the trip, or plan a recovery block afterwards to relax yourself back to neutral. For example, choose to listen to peaceful music in the car, read a book that uplifts you while you wait at reception, or plan a walk in a park afterwards. Some of those options may seem simple at first, but the power of recovery tools lies in their repetition, so the more often you employ them, the more powerful they become.

If you change your relationship to stress from avoidance to recovery, you will be more in control of how you manage your day-to-day stressors. This shift in thinking does not happen overnight, and it takes some work, but the results are profound. Just imagine all the times in a day, week, or month that you feel overwhelmed by stress. Each of these moments is an opportunity to learn to recover more efficiently, which will leave you with greater energy to spend on the activities you love.

CHAPTER SUMMARY
- Stress is unavoidable in your life, and some stress is necessary to help you achieve your goals, dreams and aspirations
- There are opportunities each day to recover from stressors—learn to identify and use them more efficiently
- Change your relationship to stress to focus on efficient recovery, and you will spend less time and energy on those stressors

HOW TO USE THIS BOOK

This book is a guide to help you create your own set of tools for taking frequent and efficient recovery breaks from stress.

This is a workbook; I hope you enjoy the read, but take the time to write down notes and fill out the forms in the book. Or better yet, photocopy the forms for future use. The intent of this book is to help you identify stress recovery tools that you already have at your disposal, and may be using unconsciously. These will range from extremely healthy and productive to potentially harmful and destructive. It will also help you to identify recovery tools that you have not tried before.

Don't worry if some of your present recovery tools are unhealthy. At the end of the chapter you will be asked to write down EVERY possible activity you do to recover or destress, no matter how silly it seems, or how rarely you do it. If you find it difficult to identify those tools you already use, there is a list in Appendix A—some may apply to you now, and some may pique your interest to try them in the future.

You will revisit your list frequently as you work through this book. Keep it nearby, and feel free to add to it as you progress. It's important to note that you will most likely favour recovery tools in one of the five divisions more than the others. When I do presentations to high performance athletes about recovery tools, they tend to create lists that are heavy on physical recovery but lack depth in other areas such as internal or spiritual recovery. However, we need at least a few interventions in each of the five areas to help us recover as quickly and efficiently as possible.

SECTIONS OF THE BOOK

This may be the smallest book you've picked up in a long time, and it's designed that way for a number of reasons. First, there are already some great books that examine, in great detail, human physiology and its relationship to stress. If you have further questions about stress and our response to it, Appendix B provides a list of great resources on the subject. Secondly, if you feel

"For fast-acting relief, try slowing down. "
– Lily Tomlin

stressed out already, you may not
want a five-hundred-page book on
stress.

Your Nervous System and
You provides an overview of the
effects of stress on your nervous
system and introduces you to the
Hypothalamus Pituitary Adrenal
axis (HPA). It's important to know
and understand, in broad terms,
the effects that stress has on our
physical bodies, and why those
responses are necessary, so that
we can appreciate all that the
system does for us on a daily basis.

The Five Divisions separates
the stressors in our lives into
five categories: physical, mental,
emotional, spiritual and internal.
Activities in this section will help
you identify how the recovery tools
you select have either a positive
or negative effect on each of the
five divisions. By the end of this
section, you will more clearly
understand how to select the
appropriate recovery method for
any given stressor, based upon
your awareness of how it will
affect each of your five divisions.

The Time Crunch helps you
identify strategies to create

recovery times in your busy life. One of the most frequent complaints about the use of recovery tools is that people don't have time for them. This section not only identifies "recovery opportunities" in daily life, but also provides a systematic approach to decrease the amount of time needed to complete a recovery method. This approach allows you to take recovery tools that would often take hours or days, and condense them to the most basic elements for daily use.

Finally, Tips and Tricks provides strategies to help you take the information you've gathered in this book and put it into use. The value of this book lies in your ability to transition this knowledge into action in your life. This section will give you those final few ideas and the encouragement to do just that.

By the end of this book, you will have identified the recovery tools that you already use, and others that you may have overlooked every day. You'll finish with real life skills and habits that can be used to redefine your relationship to stress.

"A crust eaten in peace is better than a banquet partaken in anxiety. "
– Aesop

Before you jump into the book, take five minutes and fill out **Worksheet 1: Take Stock of Your Tools**.

Try your best not to filter your ideas; instead, keep an open mind with your answers and don't worry whether you believe each method is good or bad; simply write them all down.

WORKSHEET 1:
TAKE STOCK OF YOUR TOOLS

Take a moment and write down every possible activity you use as a recovery method to destress your life. Be as broad and unfiltered as possible. If you get stuck, reference Appendix A for tools that you may not realize you use. If you run out of space, continue on a separate sheet of paper, but keep it nearby to revisit in later chapters.

If you feel stuck about whether or not an activity would count as a recovery method, ask yourself "Do I usually feel less stressed during or after this particular activity?" If the answer is yes, write it down. Preferences for certain recovery tools may change over time, so check your list frequently for any changes.

Don't worry about the second or third column until you've read The Five Divisions and The Time Crunch sections.

Activity	Divisions	Time taken

THE NERVOUS SYSTEM

This chapter will give you a basic introduction to your nervous system, so you can appreciate how your actions affect your body's response to stress. Your mood, blood pressure, dietary habits, sleep patterns, digestive movements, and so much more tie into your nervous system.

Our nervous system consists of both voluntary and involuntary branches. The voluntary nervous system is controlled by our thoughts. Actions such as moving our skeletal muscles to walk, juggle or roll our eyes at people when we're bored illustrate the voluntary nervous system at work.

In contrast, unconscious checks and balances regulate the involuntary nervous system. Hormone levels, blood pressure, heart rate and respiration are all examples of the involuntary system. It works tirelessly to keep us alive without our conscious input. It is true that we can consciously alter our heart rate or restrict our breath, but only for short periods of time. After

"Rest is not idleness, and to lie sometimes on the grass under the trees on a summer's day, listening to the murmur of water, or watching the clouds float across the sky, is by no means a waste of time."
– John Lubbock

all, you'd never get to enjoy life if you had to consciously make your heart beat every second of every day.

The involuntary nervous system has two opposite responses to stimuli—the Sympathetic Nervous System (SNS) and the Parasympathetic Nervous System (PSNS). The Sympathetic Nervous System is our fight-or-flight response; it helps us to mobilize against threats. Conversely, the Parasympathetic Nervous System is associated with rest-and-digest tendencies in the body; it helps us to grow and repair. These two systems are designed to work in unity so we can mobilize against a stressor such as a disease or threat in our environment, and then move back into a state of rest.

THE SYMPATHETIC NERVOUS SYSTEM

The Sympathetic Nervous System (SNS) is your fight-or-flight response. When activated, the SNS will mobilize your body to prepare for a possible confrontation. With your SNS engaged, your body prepares to either fight or flee from an immediate stressor. Blood pressure, heart rate and respiration rate will increase. Your body will direct blood away from digestion and towards your major muscles to prepare for fight-or-flight. The chart Effects of the Nervous System p.33 lists the effects of the sympathetic nervous system on different areas of the body. As you can see, it definitely creates a full body response.

Imagine that you have been out for dinner with your friends. You arrive home at the end of the evening and get to your front door, only to find it ajar. Immediately, your heart rate skyrockets as you ask yourself "Who could possibly be in my house?" You know you locked the door, and you can hear an intruder in a room upstairs. Your body prepares for an encounter with the stranger. Your blood pressure rises; in fact it seems like you can hear your heart beat in your ears. Your body directs blood away from your digestive organs towards your major muscle groups, and floods your bloodstream with glucose, to make sure there's enough energy in the body to feed those big muscles. This reaction in your body happens every time there's a stressor, and as we'll find out, it doesn't matter if it's real or imagined, physical or emotional. Our body will always mount a response.

Recent research indicates that our fight-or-flight response to stress is not as cut and dried as it may initially appear. The body's reaction to stress depends on whether we see that stress as a challenge or a threat. The reaction can correspond to factors such as whether or not we believe we have the necessary tools to overcome the situation. It is important to know that the way your body responds to a certain stress will in part depend on if you believe you have the necessary recovery tools to deal with that stress.

THE PARASYMPATHETIC NERVOUS SYSTEM

The Parasympathetic Nervous System (PSNS) is responsible for growth and restoration in the body. It is often called the rest-and-digest side of your nervous system, as it diverts more blood flow to the digestive organs and lowers both blood pressure and heart rate. When the SNS fires, it puts our body into a catabolic state—our body will literally break parts of itself down in order to mount a response to a stressor. The PSNS, on the other hand, is anabolic—it promotes growth and repair of damaged tissues and bodily systems.

The Parasympathetic Nervous System also plays a tremendous role in digestion, because it increases blood flow back towards digestion and absorption of food. This small shift should not be overlooked; the healthier our digestive system, the healthier our entire internal system will be. There is a growing body of evidence that links digestive distress, such as intestinal permeability, with issues throughout the body such as headaches, sleep dysregulation, anxiety and even autoimmune conditions. These issues have become a hot topic of discussion in both the mainstream and alternative healthcare community.

When you examine the chart below on the effects of the SNS

and the PSNS, it should strike you that these two sides have the exact opposite actions. This allows our body to respond to our environment and then return to normal. Usually, the body will favour the SNS over PSNS, and there's a reason for this; if you have to choose between properly digesting a donut or running from an axe murderer, you'd probably choose the latter, wouldn't you? Your nervous system agrees with you, and will quickly shift from PSNS to SNS when even remotely necessary.

N O T E S:

EFFECTS OF THE NERVOUS SYSTEM

	Sympathetic Nervous System (Fight or Flight) Parasympathetic Nervous	System (Rest and Digest)
Heart Rate	Increases	Decreases
Blood Pressure	Increases	Decreases
Digestion	Decreases blood flow to digestive organs	Increases blood flow to digestive organs
Blood Sugar	Increases glucose in blood stream	Decreases/ normalizes blood sugar levels
Respiration	Increases rate of respiration	Decreases rate of respiration

PERCEIVED VS. REAL STRESSORS

One feature of the human stress response is that we can activate it with our imagination. You may think that you're not very creative. But take a moment to imagine any bad situation that has happened, or could happen, to you or a family member. Your mind will likely take that small suggestion and conjure up all types of possible scenarios. This ability to imagine and predict future events, whether or not they have any basis in reality, is a key factor in how our SNS system becomes over activated.

Most of our stressors are perceived, as opposed to real. A perceived stress is one that we think or fixate about in the past, present or future, whether it is real or not. This is different than a stressor that demands your attention at that moment. You receive an email from your boss, asking you to meet with him the next day to discuss your role in the company. Through the night, you'll likely ruminate over what might happen the next day. In this situation, your perceived stress creates a full-blown SNS response.

"When I look back on all these worries, I remember the story of the old man who said on his deathbed that he had had a lot of trouble in his life, most of which had never happened."
– Winston Churchill

This SNS pattern will continue unless we actively break the cycle of nervous system preparation.

Some perceived stresses are valuable because they create motivation and action. It's beneficial if you're motivated to prepare thoroughly for a presentation, or if you run through a speech in your mind before you take the stage. Where we run into problems is when we are in a cycle of constant worry about future or past events; we can create the same stress response as if it actually happened in real time.

THE HYPOTHALAMUS-PITUITARY-ADRENAL AXIS AND YOU

The major way that your body responds to stressors is through the hypothalamus-pituitary-adrenal axis (HPA axis). The hypothalamus sits in the center of your brain and sends signals to the pituitary gland, directly below it, through nerve and hormone signals. You can think of the hypothalamus as the manager who tells the pituitary what to do and where to send hormones. The pituitary gland then sends out those hormones to affect the

"Stress is the trash of modern life-we all generate it but if you don't dispose of it properly, it will pile up and overtake your life."
— Danzae Pace

targeted tissue in our bodies, one of which is our adrenal glands.

The adrenal glands are located on the top of each kidney, and are responsible for the release of hormones such as epinephrine, norepinephrine (aka adrenalin and noradrenalin), and cortisol. While epinephrine is released via neuronal controls, cortisol hormones are released when the pituitary sends a messenger hormone, a little mouthful called adrenocorticotropic hormone (ACTH), through the bloodstream to the adrenal cortex.

Think about it this way; epinephrine is needed IMMEDIATELY to mobilize a sympathetic response. This is done through nerves, because it's a much faster way to get a response from the adrenals—similar to sending a text message instead of a letter in the mail. Cortisol is released to respond to longer stressors, so it's not as crucial that be is released immediately. Therefore, cortisol is regulated through hormonal controls from the pituitary that arrive at the adrenal glands through our blood.

Cortisol indirectly affects every cell in our body and performs the following functions, vital to our overall health:
- Increases blood sugar levels
- Breaks down fat into blood sugar
- Suppresses the immune system
- Mediates inflammation
- Alters short term memory storage
- Increases muscle and brain cell glucose usage

It's important to know that cortisol isn't at the same level throughout the day; it follows a circadian rhythm. This means that our levels are highest in the morning and decrease throughout the day, as shown in the following graph. There's a brilliance to this rhythm; cortisol increases blood sugar levels, but we don't want to be ready for a fight at bedtime—we want to sleep. So the nightly drop in cortisol levels allows us to fall asleep and stay asleep. We should be back to high levels in the morning, ready to take on the day.

Normal Diurnal Cortisol Range

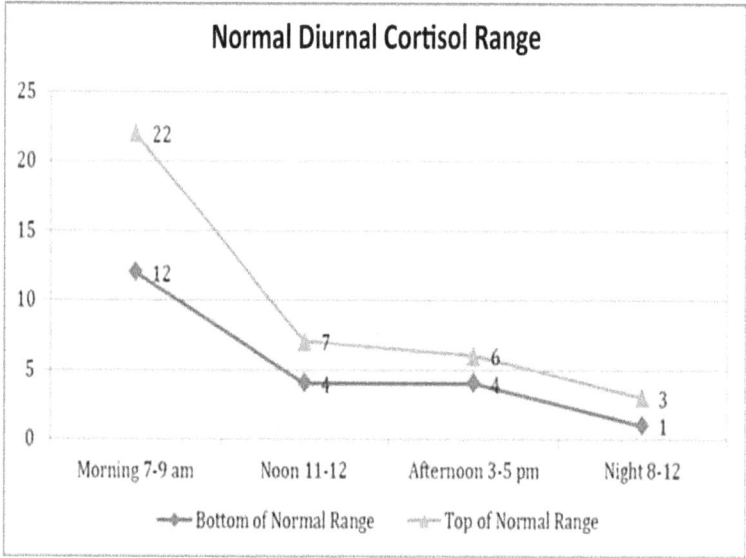

	Morning 7-9 am	Noon 11-12	Afternoon 3-5 pm	Night 8-12
Top of Normal Range	22	7	6	3
Bottom of Normal Range	12	4	4	1

— Bottom of Normal Range   — Top of Normal Range

This HPA system is constantly monitored so our body knows how much cortisol we have in circulation at any given time. If there is too much cortisol, then ACTH lowers. If there is a new stressor, ACTH increases, prompting the release of more cortisol. At least, that's how it works in a perfect system.

We have so many constant stressors that our body attempts to produce more and more cortisol to meet the demands of our lifestyles, environment and work schedules. Over time, this leads to dysregulation of the

"From time to time, one must release the grime built up inside them to to free their emotions like the ocean."
— Suzy Kassem,

HPA axis, which leaves you with elevated or depressed cortisol levels throughout the day. To put it another way, that coffee you NEED at 3 p.m. may be the result of a drastic drop in your cortisol levels in the afternoon. Or, you may be restless at night due to a release of cortisol at the wrong time, which leaves you "tired and wired." The effects of dysregulated adrenal function can show up anywhere in the body, which is why it's so important to recover between stressors and give your adrenal glands a much deserved break.

DISTRESS VS. EUSTRESS

Stress in your life can be divided into two distinct categories— distress and eustress. Distress events include stressors such as the loss of a loved one, or a divorce. Distress occurs when we are in a situation out of our control and not of our choice. These events often result in a negative experience without positive gain.

In contrast, an event that causes eustress is usually something we have chosen, even though we know there will be stress involved. Skydiving or planning a wedding will often cause stress, but you value the outcome enough to go through with it. I'm sure you can think of times in your life when you forced yourself into an activity or an environment that caused you stress, and after it was done you felt like you were on top of the world and had accomplished something special. That, my friends, is eustress.

It's important to realize that distress and eustress are different for each individual, and that they can change throughout our lives. One person may think skydiving is a eustress event and want more of it; another may find it distressful and never want to go again. Keep this in mind when you talk to friends or family about events that you find stressful; you may find that you have different opinions about what causes stress and distress.

WHAT CAN BE DONE?

So what can you do to minimize the effects of constantly living in a state of SNS domination? The

NOTES:

answer lies in how you recover
between stressors. If you choose
appropriate recovery tools between
stressors, you will minimize how
often and how long you fire your
sympathetic nervous system. This
takes time to achieve. If you are
used to a life where the sympathetic
nervous system fires relentlessly,
you will find it difficult to switch
into PSNS for rest and recovery.
The first step in recovering properly
is identifying which of the five
divisions of stress you're under, and
then picking an appropriate recovery
tool from your toolkit. With that in
mind, let's examine the five divisions
of stress and recovery.

CHAPTER SUMMARY
- Our autonomic nervous system has two
  branches, the sympathetic and the
  parasympathetic
- The sympathetic branch is our fight-or–flight
  response
- The parasympathetic branch is our rest-and-
  digest response
- Our body reacts as strongly to imaginary
  stressors as it does to real-life stressors
- Stress can be either distress or eustress; not all
  stress is bad
- We need to shift away from the fear of stress
  and begin to identify where we can recover
  better

THE FIVE DIVISIONS

PHYSICAL

Of the five divisions of recovery, the physical body is the easiest one for most people to understand. When you go for a run, lift weights, do yoga or carry boxes, you put either a positive or negative strain on your physical body.

How often have you heard a coworker, spouse, friend or stranger mention in casual conversation that they have a sore this or an achy that? Probably more often than you realize. The physical body is in a constant state of either breakdown or repair and renewal. Bone is remodelled every day of our lives, muscle and fat ratios constantly fluctuate, and our joints continuously respond to changes in our environment, footwear and posture.

Your list of recovery tools on worksheet #1 may already include movement components. Either self-directed movement like yoga, or professional therapy such as massage treatments can encourage physical recovery. For our physical body, motion is lotion;

"Conscious breathing is the best antidote to stress, anxiety and depression."
— Amit Ray

NOTES:

it increases lymphatic circulation, maintains synovial fluid levels in our joints (which keeps them moving smoothly), and increases circulation to the brain.

Lack of movement can be just as difficult on the body as too much movement. You'll know this firsthand if you've ever gone on a long road trip and stepped out of the car feeling stiff and sore.

Don't forget that recovery depends on the individual, and what is a physical recovery tool to one person may be a stress to another. If your body is used to marathons and you go for an easy twenty-minute run, it may be a physical recovery tool for you. Your body will feel refreshed, and you will have worked out some of those muscle kinks. However, if you haven't run in four years and you think you're out for a recovery run, chances are that it will be a stressor on your body and you'll end up more sore than when you began. It's important to remember your current level of activity, and select an appropriate recovery intensity from that. Don't make the mistake of thinking, "I used to run track in University so I should be able to do this easily." You'll end up a with a trip to a massage therapist where you'll have to admit, "I haven't run in twenty years, and I've just tried to run ten km." What constitutes a physical recovery for you will change, so the more honest you can be about where you are TODAY, the more efficiently you can recover.

In recent years, there's been an explosion in popularity of physical activities based on Eastern philosophy. Exercises such as Tai Chi, Chi Gong and yoga allow people to use gentle movements to work on potential recovery in all the five divisions at once. That doesn't mean you should throw this book down and rush out to buy a new pair of Lululemon pants; it's important to understand that some forms of yoga are more geared towards recovery than others. If you're unsure where to start, look for classes that are listed as gentle, yin or restorative, and go from there. Don't buy into the belief that if you don't sweat, you don't benefit. First, identify why you're motivated to try yoga, and then look for an appropriate class to help you reach that goal. If your

"The greatest weapon against stress is our ability to choose one thought over another."
– William James

goal is recovery, don't sign up for
an intense advanced yoga flow
class.

Return to your answers on Worksheet 1. Take
note of how many physical recovery tools you
have listed. If you have none, spend a few
minutes and brainstorm options that you may
have overlooked.

MENTAL

Although the mental and emotional divisions may seem similar at first, they really are two separate entities. As you'll come to understand, the emotional body deals with our reactions to people, places and events. This differs from the mental body which deals with our ability to focus on a given task, event or person. Reading a textbook may not provoke any emotions, but it might tax you mentally. An eight-hour roadtrip may not have much emotion attached to it—in fact you may love to drive—but by the end of the day you can still feel mentally fatigued and in need of recovery.

Many recovery tools that target the mental body will involve a reduction in environmental stimuli. When you meditate, take an easy walk in nature or enjoy a bath with Epsom salts and candles, you allow your brain to slow down and rest.

Our technology-laden society tends to use stimulation to "come down" after a long workday. If you commonly watch TV, play video games or spend hours on the internet, you might not enjoy as much mental recovery as you could. This may seem like a great way to relax, but it's important to keep in mind how these activities mentally tax you. True, some shows genuinely seem to numb your mind. But they still provide more sensory input than other options that don't use electronics. Some video games are deceptive brain draining activities, especially with online components that put you in realtime competition against other gamers. These activities are far from recovery tools for the brain and nervous system. They are extremely intricate and demand a high level of focus. If you play them for hours after school or work to calm yourself down, you may experience the opposite effect on your mind and nervous system.

Return to Worksheet 1 to make sure you have mental recovery options. When you analyze your answers, be sure to check whether some options involve little or no stimulation from electronics.

EMOTIONAL

Ever had a messy breakup, failed a final exam, or suffered the loss of a loved one? Chances are you've had more emotional stress, and carry more scars to prove it, than you'd ever care to admit.

If you live a life filled with activities and people you love, then you will experience emotional stress. Guaranteed. When we care about people, our work and life, we set ourselves up for emotional stress when these things change. But investing in something you care about is a crucial part of a fulfilled life. Have you ever taken a chance and told somebody that you like them—or love them? Even if they said they felt the same way about you, it was stressful to work up the courage to tell them. Have you always wanted to start a new hobby or play an instrument? Chances are those first few classes were stressful, even if it was an activity you'd dreamt about for years. Emotional stress in unavoidable. Recovery from it is in our hands. That's a powerful thought.

If you could make a complete recovery from emotional stress,

"My body needs laughter as much as it needs tears. Both are cleansers of stress."
– Mahogany SilverRain.

you would feel no sense of regret, no residual sadness or anger, and no fear that it might happen again. Of course, that is rarely the case. Usually, we carry past events with us like scars on our hearts. You probably know people whose entire identity is connected to their past emotional events. Recovery from events with an emotional component can be very difficult, but it can be done.

Tools for emotional recovery range from simple techniques such as keeping a journal, all the way to psychotherapy. Appendix A is filled with options that may help you release emotional stressors and recover more efficiently. As always, it's up to you to identify and fine-tune those ones that work best.

Return to Worksheet 1 and evaluate what recovery tools you have listed that could help you recover emotionally from stressors. Use Appendix A as a reference if you struggle to come up with options.

SPIRITUAL

Spiritual stressors refer to our relationship to concepts bigger than ourselves. Our perception of ourselves in our community, whether or not we believe our environment is safe and that it nurtures positive growth—these are examples of our spiritual side. Even the most introverted person in the world needs a sense of spiritual safety and connection to others.

For some, this will include religious beliefs and practices. Religion offers a framework that can help people feel connected to their community, and gives them a sense that they are a part of a greater picture.

It's important to take time to help our legs recover from a run, or our brains recover from a test, but we also need ways to help us recover a sense of safety, humility, and a belief that we belong. This area of recovery is often overlooked, although it impacts our quality of life as much as any other area. Think about it; if you believe your environment is unsafe, how will that affect

"The stressful life leads to neglect of spirituality and wellness."
– Lailah Gifty Akita

your life on a day-to-day basis? If you believe that nobody cares about you, how likely are you to use the available resources in your community? These maladies of the soul require immediate and continual attention. Thankfully, if you open your eyes to them, recovery tools for spiritual stressors can be found in many places.

People join recreational sport leagues, churches, social groups or book clubs partly for the sense of community that comes with spending time with people who have similar interests. Then, if the people in the group are kind and welcoming, there is no end to the possibilities for spiritual recovery. Some people prefer a hike and time spent in nature. For others, it's coffee with friends, or the weekly ritual of wings every Wednesday. All of these activities have the potential to provide spiritual recovery.

So how do you know if you've found a method that works for you? When you leave the group or activity with a greater sense of happiness, even though there is no tangible reason for it—you've found spiritual recovery. You might feel humbled, or as though you have a greater connection to the people you've just spent time with, and you may feel a sense of connection to your environment as well. One reason that yoga centers have popped up all over the country is that they usually provide a welcome centre for people to meet. I know many knowledgeable yoga practitioners who could easily develop rich home practices, but they choose to practice in their favourite yoga studio. They enjoy the spiritual benefit of day-to-day community connections.

Return to Worksheet 1, and evaluate your answers to make sure you have recovery tools for spiritual stressors. Additional ideas can be found in Appendix A.

INTERNAL

The internal body is composed of all the wonderful magic that goes on inside you that you take for granted until something begins to fail. Blood pH, food sensitivities, intestinal permeability, intestinal parasites and hormone levels are all the internal body at work. These internal systems fluctuate constantly as they respond to environmental changes inside your body. These conditions are dependant on both internal and external factors, so the conditions outside your body will affect the quality of your internal environment.

Symptoms associated with internal stressors affect virtually every part of our body. Headaches, energy crashes in the afternoon, constipation, diarrhoea, foggy brain, acne, irritability, anxiety, sleep difficulties, decreased motivation, muscle aches and joint pain—the list seems endless. Clearly it's worth the effort to keep our internal system as happy as possible to resolve some of these issues, or to avoid them entirely.

For many people, these internal stressors are the hardest to conceptualize. We don't get much information about them until we go for lab tests. Unless you have experienced difficulties with pregnancies or recently gone through menopause, you probably don't know how much estrogen or progesterone your body produces. Many people never realize that they suffer from food sensitivities that cause symptoms elsewhere in their body. To look closely at our internal systems, we need a qualified healthcare provider who is trained to run and analyze tests. These tests can help us understand our internal environment, so we can find ways to heal from the inside out. Look for a practitioner who not only interprets tests, but who searches for clinical correlations between those results and any symptoms that you have. There has been a substantial growth in the number of providers trained in Integrative Medicine, Functional Diagnostic Nutrition and Naturopathy. These professionals can be great resources to identify and treat internal stressors.

NOTES:

""It was after I first began to uplift my thoughts a bit that my cravings for junk food started to dissipate. I did not connect the two at that time. First, I simply noticed that I didn't need to sleep so much. It took a while before I realized that in addition to my improved energy level, there was a direct correlation between chewing on mental garbage and putting garbage in my mouth."
— Holly Mosier

Internal recovery tools take the form of dietary changes, avoidance of environmental toxins, supplements and other tools that affect more than one of the five divisions. Meditation is a great example of a method that is often seen as mental or emotional recovery, but can also positively affect your internal environment.

Return to your answers on Worksheet 1. Note which recovery tools you listed that would help your internal systems recover from stress more efficiently.

NET GAINS AND LOSSES

By now, you've identified various recovery tools that you use in your life. But you've probably noticed that some of these tools have a positive impact on one area of your body and a negative impact on another.

It's just as important to understand how your recovery tools might impact you negatively, as it is to understand how they impact you positively. If you fully understand how each of the five divisions is impacted by the decisions you make, you're in a better position to pick those tools that will give you the highest degree of overall recovery.

If you're a person who enjoys a glass of wine as a recovery tool at the end of a busy day, don't despair; I'm not suggesting that you never drink again, or that you must live the life of a monk. Instead, when you choose to have drinks with friends, be aware of the effects it will have on the different divisions of your body and the recovery you'll need over the next hour, day or week. Do you

"How beautiful it is to do nothing, and then to rest afterward."
– Spanish proverb

have a big presentation at work the next day? Maybe you'll choose water over wine, because you know how wine will make your physical body feel the next day. On a cruise through the Caribbean, spending your days asleep by the poolside? Then maybe you choose to let yourself have more fun. The important difference is the consciousness behind your choice of recovery method. Identify the positive and negative effects on your body, and you will better understand why you choose those actions.

Take a moment and return to the list of recovery tools you listed in Worksheet 1. Note which tools have a positive, negative, or neutral effect on each of the five divisions. Give a +1 if the method helps that area, a -1 if it is detrimental, and a 0 if it's neutral. Remember to score them in the context of how well they let you recover. Certain physical activities like a long run might actually score -1 for the physical body, but be a +1 for mental or emotional recovery if you know that you return from a long run and feel calm, refreshed and more mentally at peace. As you go through your list and score your recovery responses, ask yourself "how does this make me feel during and after the activity?"

CHAPTER SUMMARY

- We can divide our stressors and recovery into five sections; physical, mental, emotional, spiritual and internal
- Your recovery tools are individualized; some that work for you might not work for your friends or spouses, and that's okay
- Some recovery tools will help you across more than one of the stress divisions
- Some recovery tools will be positive in one area and negative in others
- Understand why you use a certain recovery tool; it's as important as the method itself
- Recovery tool preferences change over time, so review your list of tools frequently

"If the problem can be solved why worry? If the problem cannot be solved worrying will do you no good."
— Śāntideva

THE TIME CRUNCH

One of the biggest issues that people complain about is a lack of time. Time is money, time is precious, and time ticks away whether we want it to or not. So why should anybody spend precious time on their recovery? You may think, "Those ideas sound nice for a single person in their twenties, but I have three kids to look after!" Trust me, you too can, and deserve to, recover from your daily stressors. But if you want to recover better, the first step is to understand that there are different recovery tools for different times in your day, week or year.

How often have you experienced this situation; it's a month away from your annual vacation to somewhere hot and peaceful, but where you are now is cold and chaotic. You wonder if your whole company will come apart if you take two weeks off. So you put your head down, work as hard as you can for that last month before your trip, and all the time you think, "I just have to get to my vacation...then I'll relax." The last week of work feels like a month, and the last day feels like a whole week, until finally you're on vacation.

And you get sick.

"How the heck could this happen to me? I worked so hard to get here, this isn't fair!"

But it is fair.

Your body thinks it's fair whether you like it or not. You've worked harder than ever at your job, while neglecting your recovery in the weeks prior to your vacation. Your body is now similar to that of an amateur runner who has just crossed the finish line of their first marathon—battered, bruised and ready to collapse.

Now contrast the above story with a different premise. You are a month away from your planned vacation to somewhere hot and peaceful, but at home life is cold and chaotic. You're excited about your trip, but you need to get work done before you leave, without destroying yourself in the process. So you put in time at work, but stick to your exercise program, still choose to eat healthy food and cook real meals at home. How often do you neglect healthy food choices for the last four days before a trip because you don't want to deal with leftovers and

> *"Stress is caused by being 'here' but wanting to be 'there.'*
> *– Eckhart Tolle*

dishes? You still meet your friend for coffee, and you and your spouse continue to make time to go for a walk or read before bed. The last week of work before your vacation feels like a week; maybe at most like the Beatles' song "Eight Days a Week," and the last day feels like a busy day. You go on your vacation and don't get sick. You enjoy the time to recharge fully, and return to work refreshed and grateful for the escape.

Sound impossible? Maybe you should examine your approach to recovery. To understand how recovery works on a day-to-day basis(drum roll please...), you need enough recovery tools in your toolbox to recover in thirty seconds, five minutes, fifteen minutes, an hour, a half-day and a day. And you need to know WHY you use these tools, and WHEN you can use them.

Here's an example. As a massage therapist my hands and arms are, in many ways, the breadwinners in my household. To keep them in good condition, I need recovery tools that work in each of those time opportunities. So, if I have thirty seconds while

I wait at a traffic light, I stretch a forearm. Take a moment to think about this, because the beauty is in the simplicity. I use that part of my daily commute to recover, whereas most people think about their commute as another source of stress. It's also a time that is consistent in my life, which makes it more likely that I will stretch while going both to and from work. Make no mistake, these little opportunities add up over the long run, far more than if I blocked off one hour every week to stretch my arms. I'm not sure I could make it that long without these tiny opportunities for physical recovery.

If I have five to fifteen minutes, I can do contrast baths or self-massage my forearms. If I have an hour, I get a massage from another therapist. Finally, if I have a half or full day off work, I can rest my forearms more completely if I consciously avoid certain activities that would tire them out. I understand that it's not a rest day for my arms if I play video games or type on the computer for hours. This is one example of how I've redefined and rethought my recovery with fantastic results.

To recover more efficiently, you must take advantage of the small slots in your day that you can use to get back into a state of relaxation and activate your Parasympathetic Nervous System. The more you practice, the easier it becomes to drop back into that state of mind. So don't give up on a method after only one try; give it a few weeks of genuine effort and you'll find it becomes more and more valuable.

HOW TO CREATE A TRIGGER

If you've identified recovery tools that work for you, but you have no idea what to do for smaller daily opportunities, don't despair. You can trim any recovery method into smaller key segments to get at least a portion of the benefits of the activity. This may seem complicated at first, but with a little thought and creativity it can be done easily.

I love a gentle hike in the mountains as a form of physical, emotional, mental and spiritual recovery. When I finish my hike, I feel rested, calm, and more connected to my environment than when I began. Unfortunately, I can't do this everyday, unless I want to lose my house and my job.

Let's identify the key components of this activity—the sights of nature, the sounds (or lack thereof), the smells (of the woods) and gentle physical movement. If I want to create a recovery trigger with those features in mind, I can find a park near my work and walk there on my lunch break. Or I can upload a slideshow of hikes I've done onto my computer, use headphones to play nature sounds, and recapture some of the benefits of a hike, in five minutes or less, while sitting at my desk. Would I prefer going outside for a hike? Definitely. But I can recreate elements of a longer recovery method in a matter of minutes or seconds, which then allows me to integrate them seamlessly into my day.

Take a moment, go back to your list of recovery options, and select one of the five major forms. Then ask yourself, "Do I have options for different time demands?" Don't be surprised if you find this difficult at first, I know I did when I started this process. If you need help, check Appendix A for suggestions of different tools. But I encourage you to do that only after you've really given it some thought. It's important to challenge your brain to question what you do to recover and why. This will help you come up with creative solutions that will work with your life.

CHAPTER SUMMARY

- There are tiny opportunities to recover every day; at red lights, in the elevator, at the office, etc.
- It's important to have recovery tools that can be accomplished in different time restraints, from thirty seconds to several days
- Recovery tools get more efficient over time; there's power in repetition
- You can create a trigger to drop quickly into a state of recovery if you identify the key features of the recovery tool you enjoy, and build them into shorter timeframes

TIPS AND TRICKS

By this point in the book, you should have more resources available to you than ever before. You probably think that you're ready to go out there and take on the world, and you are. Here are a final few tips and tricks that can help you transition seamlessly into more efficient recovery.

CHOOSE RECOVERY TOOLS THAT ARE RIGHT FOR YOU

Just as you have a unique fingerprint, you have a unique set of recovery tools that are ideal to help you recover as efficiently as possible. It's important to remember that this is your journey; there's no quick list of activities or exercises that works for everybody every time. In fact, this is where we get ourselves into trouble. We believe we should do what we see our friends do to recover. Certain practices create positive responses in MOST people—but not all people.

Keep an open mind when you try new tools or activities for recovery.

"Stress level: extreme. It's like she was a jar with the lid screwed on too tight, and inside the jar were pickles, angry pickles, and they were fermenting, and about to explode."
— Fiona Wood

Remember, one factor that causes stress is a new situation. Ask yourself, "How do I feel, and is it from the activity or the newness of this situation?" If a friend or colleague tells you what they do to recover, see it as advice, not gospel. Understand that it may work wonders for them, but not necessarily for you.

When you try a new method, try it multiple times. There is strength in repetition, and the more you practice a recovery tool, the more benefit you should see from it. Each time you use a recovery tool, it creates a quicker and more efficient response from your body.

When you try a new recovery method, fill out a section in **Worksheet #2:** New Recovery Strategies. Note what the activity was, your recovery goals, and how you felt. Were you nervous after the first time, but great once you got the hang of it? Or did you notice that you felt no change after five or six times? How did it make you feel before, during and after the activity? Were you cxcitcd to go back? Do this four or five times. These questions will provide you with a personal roadmap to your recovery plan; only you can answer them, and you'll gain the knowledge necessary to choose the right method for the right time.

One final word on experimentation with new recovery tools; quantity does not trump quality. In fact, often the reverse is true. Think about it this way; you need at least one recovery method for each of the five categories so you can recover as efficiently as possible. You also need tools that can be done in a short time, and some that may take longer. What you don't need are three hundred different recovery tools that you don't use. Try new tools, but don't obsess over what else may be out there. Instead, focus first on your recovery method cheat sheet; make sure you have activities for each of the five categories and different time restraints. Then, if you have time and energy to nose around in new activities, you can experiment, knowing that you can fall back on the solid foundation of your core set of recovery tools.

MAKE A CHEAT SHEET

You have written down all of your recovery tools on **Worksheet #1** and plan on reviewing it occasionally. Now make a "recovery cheat sheet" from a small piece of paper or an old business card. List your favourite recovery options for thirty seconds, five minutes, fifteen and thirty minutes. Be sure to have a few different options that address the different forms of recovery. Keep this cheat sheet in your wallet or purse as a reminder of your options for quick recovery opportunities. These are the recovery chances that we often miss, but they will change our relationship with stress.

Once you've made your cheat sheet, review your list at least once every three months. It won't take long to look at your list to see if you still use the same tools, or if there are others that you have found since you last checked in. Feel free to adjust as often as necessary. Remember, the quality of the list, not the quantity of recovery tools listed, will ensure the best long-term success.

INVOLVE OTHERS

You'll be amazed how many different recovery tools are right at your fingertips. One of the best ways to learn about them is to involve your friends and family in the conversation. Don't be afraid to act like a recovery detective; if you know someone who seems to have their ducks in a row, ask them what tools they use to recover. Don't be surprised if they don't have an immediate answer. People rarely discuss "recovery tools," and may struggle to put into words what tools they use and why they use them. Some people will give you a blank stare the first time you breach the subject, but will come back to the topic a few days later and say, "I realized I do... to recover; I just never thought about it."

When you involve other people in the discussion about recovery tools, you open yourself up to learn about other recovery options that you never even thought of. If you ask five people who each use five different tools, you have tapped into the collective knowledge of the group and increased your chances to find recovery tools that might be right for you.

Also, when your friends and family are aware of your recovery tools, you create external accountability. If you have a rough day or go through a negative time in your life, you have people who can remind you to take time for yourself to recover more efficiently.

Finally, if you open up the discussion to those around you, it encourages them to recover more efficiently as well. Whether your friends and family are aware of it, they all try to recover. If they grab a cup of coffee, it's their attempt to recover energy that just isn't there that morning. Do they nap on the couch? Same premise. The power lies in the intent behind the action, so the more you understand what drives you to choose a certain method, the more you can identify those that are positive, and those which won't serve you in the long run. Just talk to people about recovery; those conversations and reflection could improve their own recovery.

GIVE YOURSELF PERMISSION

Recovery from daily stressors is one of the most valuable habits you can cultivate for your overall health. The positive effects overlap into every aspect of your life, from your energy levels to your interactions with people around you. If you don't recover properly, you'll struggle to reach your full potential. So give yourself PERMISSION to take time to recover.

This can seem impossible at first; we tend to believe that if we don't oversee activities at the office or the home that the wheels will fall off in five minutes or less. But realize that if you operate at your best, you may not need to run at full capacity at all times. You'll have more energy when it is truly needed.

When you give yourself permission to recover, you validate the importance of your health. Although it may seem selfish at first, understand that it will yield more energy and healthier interactions with the people you love. This can be a

"Its not stress that kills us, it is our reaction to it."
– Hans Selye

huge mental hurdle for people. Often, we believe that if we don't sacrifice for others, we are selfish. This couldn't be farther from the truth. If you struggle with this, then use Worksheet #3: Identify the Why, and write down all the ways you COULD be better to those around you. Maybe if you had more energy you'd do the laundry more frequently. Or, if you weren't so exhausted, you wouldn't be as quick to get angry with your children or spouse. If you could take a small amount of time each day to recover, how might it help with those issues? If you took a 10-15 minute nap, would it give you the extra energy needed to get through another three hours of productivity? That seems like a pretty good return on the time invested in recovery. If you had a small window of time to relax with a cup of tea, could you recover enough to laugh a little at the chaos of your family life? If so, then isn't it worth it, not only for your own recovery, but also for the overall health of your family? Understand this; for you to recover properly and be the best person you can be, you MUST give yourself permission to make your recovery a priority.

Once you've identified WHY you need to recover more efficiently and more frequently, involve your spouse, friends or children into the conversation. After all, you'll need their support. If you've already written down and identified how your recovery time will make you a better husband, wife or parent, it will be easier to stand your ground and convince those around you how this information will help. Be firm but flexible; offer up a one-month trial to show how proper recovery can help you, and in turn help the loved ones around you.

VALUE YOUR RECOVERY

Value your recovery time as much as you value your business life, family commitments and social obligations, or it will be the first part of your life to fall off when times get tough—and that's when you need it the most. This is one of the most common issues people run up against when they attempt to make positive changes in their lives; they start off strong, but then the wheels fall off when the stress begins to build up.

"When I take a break, even just a brief one, the creative energy flows in. Only then do I have anything of value to share with others. Once I recognized this, I stopped feeling guilty about taking time for myself."
— Holly Mosier

You acknowledge the importance of your recovery when you

schedule recovery times into your calendar. Oddly, we often reserve our calendars for business activities and maybe the annual vacation. Prioritize your recovery times in your calendar, because those commitments that don't get in your calendar will take a backseat to those that are written down. For better or for worse, our calendar subtly dictates where we put our energy and where our priorities lie.

BE CREATIVE

This book gives ideas and suggestions about how to recover more efficiently and frequently, but it is by no means the end of the conversation. There are a million different ways to recover, and you are unique. Don't be afraid to try a new activity to see how it helps you recover. Then you will know whether it is a tool you can use for years to come, or one that doesn't work for you.

I find it difficult to carve out recovery time for myself when I'm at home; I think that if I don't do the laundry tonight the world will end, or that the dishes simply demand my attention right now. Sound familiar?

I've discovered other creative ways to use my daily commute for personal recovery. On a sunny day, I'll park further away, and walk to and from my office. Or I'll stop at a coffee shop on my commute and take ten minutes alone with a cup of tea. I arrive at home or work feeling more relaxed, because I've already taken some time to come down from any stressors in my day. I can be more present for my wife than if I race home and arrived frazzled and frustrated.

Creativity goes a long way when it comes to daily recovery. If you come up against a wall, ask yourself and people around for a solution that might work for the situation. You'll be surprised how often one comes up.

FINAL THOUGHTS

With the speed of technology and our lifestyles, it's difficult to stay grounded. But if you incorporate the practice of recovery into your life, you will be able to weather the storm more efficiently and return to normal more quickly than you ever imagined.

If you've done the worksheets, you're more than halfway there. Implement your strategies, and see how good you can feel when you take time to recover from the many stresses, large and small, that build up in your life. Never forget that you are responsible for your health and wellness, and the greatest gift you can give the people you love is your full, undivided self. This is only possible if you take time to care for yourself. It's not selfish; it's a gift to all those people around you. The gift of being the best you that you can be.

WORKSHEET #2: NEW RECOVERY STRATEGIES

Are you ready to try a new recovery strategy? Use this sheet to track how you feel before, during and afterwards, so you'll know how it affects you. Be sure to note if it's the first, second or third time you try a given activity, so that you can identify how your reaction to it may change.

When you fill out how you feel before, during and after, check in with your body and see if you can identify how each of the five divisions feel. Fill out the "During" section after you've completed the activity.

Date	Activity	Before	During	After

WORKSHEET #3: IDENTIFY YOUR "WHY"

In **Column A,** write down the ways you think you could be better to yourself or those around you. Perhaps you wish you had more energy to do laundry, were less judgmental of your spouse or even that you weren't as exhausted when you got home from work.

Then fill out **Column B** with any of the five recovery divisions that might help you to be better in your **Column A** list. If there is more than one recovery tool that would help with an issue in **Column A**, then write all of them in **Column B**.

Finally, in **Column C,** brainstorm recovery solutions that work for all the different divisions identified in **Column B**. This process, where you identify an area in your life where you would like improvement, then come up with solutions, helps you to understand that you are not selfish when you take the time for proper recovery. In fact, this exercise can help you be a better spouse, worker or parent. Note how long the activity took in **Column D**.

COLUMN A: How could you be better?	COLUMN B: What divisions do you need to recover?	COLUMN C: What recovery tools might help?	COLUMN D: Time taken

APPENDIX A: RECOVERY TOOLS

This list was compiled through discussions with friends, family, and clients to serve as an example of different ways people recover. Some are more productive than others, but its important to identify all the tools you use, whether they will serve you in the long run or not.

Acupuncture	Call a friend	Craft	Yoga
Drink alcohol	Drink coffee	Eat junk food	Email a friend
Garden	Go out for coffee	Have sex	Journal
Lift weights	Listen to music	Get a massage	Needlework
Paint	Poetry	Read a book	Reflexology
Reiki	Sew	Skype a friend	Sleep
Take a nap	Text a friend	Volunteer	Make wine or beer
Write	Star gaze	Make a small animation	Spend time with family
Photography	Go for a Picnic	Go for a walk	Spend time with a pet
Play video games	Play card games	Play board games	Crochet
Go for a car ride	Go for a run	Knit	Meditate
Pottery	Send a letter	Smoke	Woodwork
Hike	Spend time alone	Blog	

APPENDIX B: RECOMMENDED READING

BOOKS

McGonigal, K, 2015. The Upside of Stress: Why Stress is Good for You, and How to Get Good at It. 2015, Penguin Publishing Group
Sapolsky, R, 2004. Why Zebras Don't get Ulcers: The Acclaimed Guide to Stress, Stress-Related Diseases and Coping. Henry Holt and Co.
Waitzkin, J, 2007.The Art of Learning: An Inner Journey to Optimal Performance. Free Press.

PODCASTS

Art Of Charm
Psychology of Change with Adam Gilbert
Emotional First Aid with Guy Winch
Ruthless Meditation with Tony Stubblebine
Start with Why with Simon Sinek
Mastering Happiness with Gretchen Rubin

Underground Wellness
#242 Heidi Hanna: 5 Stress Busting Strategies for Busy People
#308 Dr. Alan Christianson: The Adrenal Reset Diet
#326 Gretchen Rubin: 8 Strategies for Creating Habits that Stick
#348 Reed Davis: Final Episode

*9 780995 166301 *